Diabetes cookbook for adults

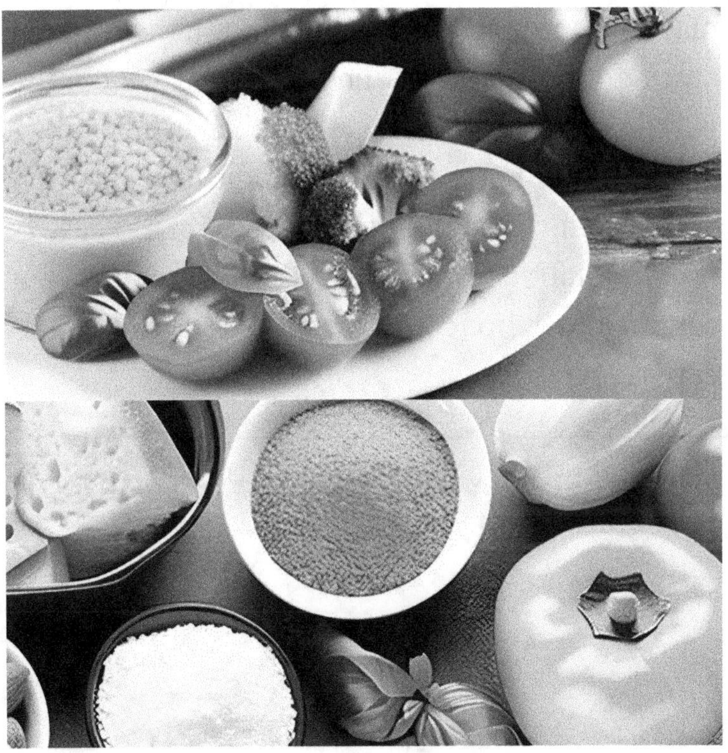

Dr. Janet Damico

TABLE OF CONTENTS

Chapter one

Chapter Two

Chapter Three

Chapter four

Chapter five

Chapter Six

Introduction

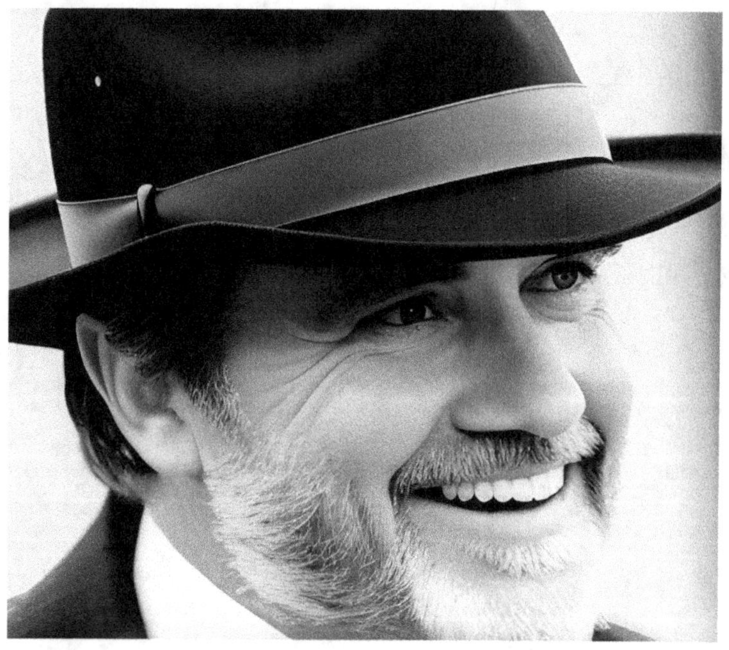

As a diabetic person, I fought for years to keep a balanced diet. I liked eating and had a hard time giving up the things I enjoyed. But as my health began to decline, I knew I needed to make a change.

That's when I found the "Diabetes Cookbook for Adults." I was hesitant at first, but after going through the recipes and ideas for a diabetes-friendly diet, I felt encouraged. Maybe I could eat excellent cuisine and yet control my diabetes.

I decided to give it a try and began food planning for the week ahead. The first morning, I made myself a low-carb omelet with vegetables and cheese. It was so filling and flavorful, I couldn't believe it was diabetes-friendly. And the greatest part? My blood sugar levels stayed constant.

As the week proceeded, I attempted other dishes from the booklet, such as grilled salmon with roasted veggies and quinoa and black bean salad. I even got creative and created a spinach and feta-filled chicken breast for my family, who liked it.

One of my favorite things about the cookbook was that it featured snacks and sweets, which I thought I'd have to give up totally. But instead, I indulged in dark chocolate and nut clusters and fruit and yogurt parfait guilt-free.

As the weeks moved into months, I started to notice a major change in my health. My blood sugar levels were regularly constant, and I had more energy than I had in years. I also dropped weight, which was an extra plus.

But it wasn't just about the physical changes. I felt powerful and in charge of my diabetes for the first time. I no longer felt like I was at the mercy of my sickness. Instead, I had a tool in the "Diabetes Cookbook for Adults" that helped me control it.

Now, years later, I still turn to the cookbook when I need ideas for healthy and tasty recipes. And I constantly suggest it to everyone I know who's dealing with diabetes control.

Looking back, I understand that my road to a better living wasn't simple. But the "Diabetes Cookbook for Adults" made it a whole lot easier. It offered me the skills and recipes I needed to take charge of my health and enhance my life. And for that, I'll always be thankful.

Chapter one

What is diabetes?

Diabetes is a chronic condition that affects the way your body uses glucose, the major source of energy for your cells. Glucose originates from the food you consume, and it is delivered by your blood to your cells, where it is utilized for energy. However, for glucose to enter your cells, it needs a hormone called insulin.

In persons with diabetes, their body is either unable to make enough insulin or unable to utilize the insulin it produces adequately. This leads to excessive amounts of glucose in the blood, which may create a range of health concerns over time.

There are three basic forms of diabetes: type 1, type 2, and gestational diabetes.

Type 1 diabetes is an autoimmune illness that commonly develops in infancy or adolescence. In type 1 diabetes, the immune system mistakenly attacks and destroys the cells in the pancreas that produce insulin. This implies that persons with type 1 diabetes need to receive insulin injections or use an insulin pump to maintain their blood sugar levels.

Type 2 diabetes is the most prevalent type of diabetes, accounting for roughly 90% of cases. Type 2 diabetes is normally diagnosed in maturity, however, it is becoming increasingly frequent in children and teens. In type 2 diabetes, the body becomes resistant to the effects of insulin, which means that glucose is unable to enter cells properly. As a consequence, the pancreas may generate more insulin to attempt to compensate, but over time, it may not be able to keep up, resulting in high blood sugar levels.

Gestational diabetes is a kind of diabetes that develops during pregnancy. It happens when the hormones released during pregnancy make it difficult for the body to utilize insulin adequately. In most instances, gestational diabetes goes away after the baby is delivered, but it might raise the chance of getting type 2 diabetes later in life.

Various risk factors might raise your probability of having diabetes. These include:

Family history: If you have a close relative with diabetes, your chance of having the condition is increased.
Obesity: Being overweight or obese increases your chance of acquiring type 2 diabetes.
Inactivity: A sedentary lifestyle might raise your chance of acquiring type 2 diabetes.
Age: The chance of acquiring diabetes rises as you become older.
Ethnicity: Certain ethnic groups, such as African Americans, Hispanics, and Native Americans, have a greater chance of having diabetes.

Symptoms of diabetes may include:

Frequent urination
Excessive thirst
Fatigue
Blurred vision
Slow-healing sores or illnesses
Tingling or numbness in the hands or feet

If you are experiencing any of these symptoms, it is crucial to consult a healthcare practitioner for a diagnosis. Diabetes may be diagnosed with a blood test that checks your blood sugar levels.

Managing diabetes takes a lifetime commitment to maintaining good practices. This involves adopting a balanced diet, getting regular exercise, monitoring your blood sugar levels, and taking medication as advised by your healthcare expert. With good control, individuals with diabetes may live long, healthy lives and lower their risk of developing problems such as heart disease, kidney damage, and blindness.

Why is nutrition crucial for controlling diabetes?

Diet has a significant part in regulating diabetes. When you have diabetes, your body is unable to digest glucose properly, which means that your blood sugar levels might grow excessively high. By selecting healthy food choices and adopting a balanced diet, you may help manage your blood sugar levels and lower your chance of developing issues associated with diabetes.

One of the most essential components of treating diabetes with food is reducing your carbohydrate consumption. Carbohydrates are a kind of food that your body breaks down into glucose, which is subsequently utilized for energy. However, when you have diabetes, your body may not be able to process carbohydrates properly, which can cause your blood sugar levels to spike. By controlling your carbohydrate consumption and selecting nutritious, complex carbs like whole grains, fruits, and vegetables, you may help manage your blood sugar levels.

Another key part of treating diabetes with a diet is lowering your consumption of sugar and processed foods. Foods that are rich in sugar may cause your blood sugar levels to jump, and they can also contribute to weight gain, which is a risk factor for type 2 diabetes. Processed meals may also be heavy in salt, which might raise your chance of developing high blood pressure, another consequence of diabetes.

In addition to reducing your carbohydrate and sugar consumption, it is crucial to pick appropriate sources of protein and fat. Protein and fat may help you feel full and satisfied, and they can also help manage your blood sugar levels. Choosing healthy sources of protein such as lean meats, fish, beans, and tofu will help you achieve your nutritional requirements without causing your blood sugar levels to jump. Healthy sources of fat like avocados, almonds, and olive oil may also help manage your blood sugar levels and minimize your chance of getting heart disease, another consequence of diabetes.

It is also crucial to pay attention to portion sizes while treating diabetes via food. Overeating may cause your blood sugar levels to jump, and it can also lead to weight gain. By regulating your portion sizes and eating frequent, balanced meals throughout the day, you may help manage your blood sugar levels and maintain a healthy weight.

In addition to adopting appropriate eating choices, it is also crucial to keep hydrated while controlling diabetes. Drinking water and other sugar-free liquids may help manage your blood sugar levels and minimize your risk of dehydration, which can be a consequence of diabetes.

Overall, nutrition plays a key part in treating diabetes. By selecting healthy food choices and maintaining a balanced diet, you may help manage your blood sugar levels, minimize your chance of developing issues associated with diabetes, and maintain a healthy weight. If you have diabetes, it is vital to collaborate with your healthcare provider and a qualified dietitian to design a meal plan that fulfills your nutritional requirements and suits your lifestyle. With the appropriate diet and lifestyle choices, you can live a long, healthy life with diabetes.

Key elements of a diabetes-friendly diet

When it comes to controlling diabetes, adopting a balanced, diabetic-friendly diet is key. A diabetic-friendly diet should concentrate on regulating blood sugar levels, keeping a healthy weight, and lowering the risk of problems associated with diabetes. Here are some key principles of a diabetes-friendly diet:

Focus on complex carbs: Complex carbohydrates are a significant source of energy for the body, but they are also broken down more slowly than simple carbohydrates, which may help manage blood sugar levels. Examples of complex carbs include entire grains, legumes, and vegetables.

Limit simple carbs: Simple carbohydrates are broken down rapidly by the body and may induce rises in blood sugar levels. Sugary beverages, candy, and processed meals are examples of simple carbs that should be minimized in a diabetes-friendly diet.

Choose lean proteins: Lean proteins are an essential element of a diabetes-friendly diet, since they may help manage blood sugar levels and induce satiety. Examples of lean proteins include chicken, fish, tofu, and beans.

Incorporate healthy fats: Healthy fats, such as those found in nuts, seeds, and avocado, can help reduce inflammation in the body and protect against heart disease, which is a common complication of diabetes.

Eat a variety of fruits and vegetables: Fruits and vegetables are rich in vitamins, minerals, and fiber, which may help manage blood sugar levels and enhance overall health. However, it is important to be mindful of the carbohydrate content of certain fruits and vegetables and to eat them in moderation.

Monitor portion sizes: Eating too much of any meal, including nutritious ones, may cause blood sugar levels to surge and lead to weight gain. It is crucial to regulate portion sizes and eat meals that are balanced and fulfilling.

Stay hydrated: Drinking plenty of water and other sugar-free beverages can help regulate blood sugar levels and prevent dehydration, which can be a complication of diabetes.

Work with a healthcare professional and registered dietitian: Managing diabetes may be challenging, and it is vital to collaborate with a healthcare provider and a qualified dietitian to establish a meal plan that matches your particular nutritional requirements and suits your lifestyle.

By following the five basic principles of a diabetic-friendly diet, persons with diabetes may help manage blood sugar levels, maintain a healthy weight, and lower the risk of problems associated with diabetes. It is essential to remember that treating diabetes via nutrition is not a one-size-fits-all strategy, and patients should collaborate with their healthcare provider and registered dietitian to build a tailored meal plan that suits their particular requirements.

Tips for meal planning and preparation

Meal planning and preparation are crucial components of controlling diabetes. Here are some tips for meal planning and preparation that can help individuals with diabetes maintain a healthy diet:

Plan: Take time each week to plan out meals and snacks for the next week. This may help ensure that meals are balanced and healthful and can also save time and money.

Keep a well-stocked pantry: Keep healthy staples on hand, such as whole grains, legumes, and canned or frozen fruits and vegetables. This might make it simpler to prepare nutritious meals and snacks on short notice.

Use a food scale and measuring cups: Portion management is vital for controlling diabetes, and using a food scale and measuring cups may help ensure that quantities are correct and consistent.

Batch cook: Consider batch-cooking dishes and freezing them in individual quantities. This may make it simpler to have nutritious meals on hand for busy days or times when cooking is not feasible.

Make use of kitchen gadgets: Using kitchen appliances, such as a slow cooker, may make meal preparation simpler and more effective. For example, slow cooker dishes may be made ahead of time and allowed to cook all day, making it simple to have a nutritious supper ready when you come home from work.

Experiment with different recipes: Eating a healthy diet does not have to be boring. Experimenting with various dishes and tastes may make healthy eating more pleasurable and help avoid boredom.

Be careful of restaurant meals: Eating out may be tough for those with diabetes since many restaurant meals are rich in calories, fat, and sugar. When eating out, be mindful of portion sizes and choose restaurants that offer healthy options.

Involve family and friends: Getting family and friends involved in meal planning and preparation can make it more enjoyable and can also provide additional support and accountability.

Consider working with a licensed dietitian: Registered dietitians may give tailored nutrition advice and can help patients with diabetes design a meal plan that matches their particular nutritional requirements and suits their lifestyle.

By following these suggestions for meal planning and preparation, persons with diabetes may help ensure that they are eating a nutritious, balanced diet that satisfies their nutritional requirements and promotes their overall health. It is essential to remember that treating diabetes with food is a lifetime effort, and patients should engage with their healthcare provider and registered dietitian to build a meal plan that matches their particular requirements and suits their lifestyle.

Chapter Two

Breakfast Ideas

Low-carb omelet with vegetables and cheese

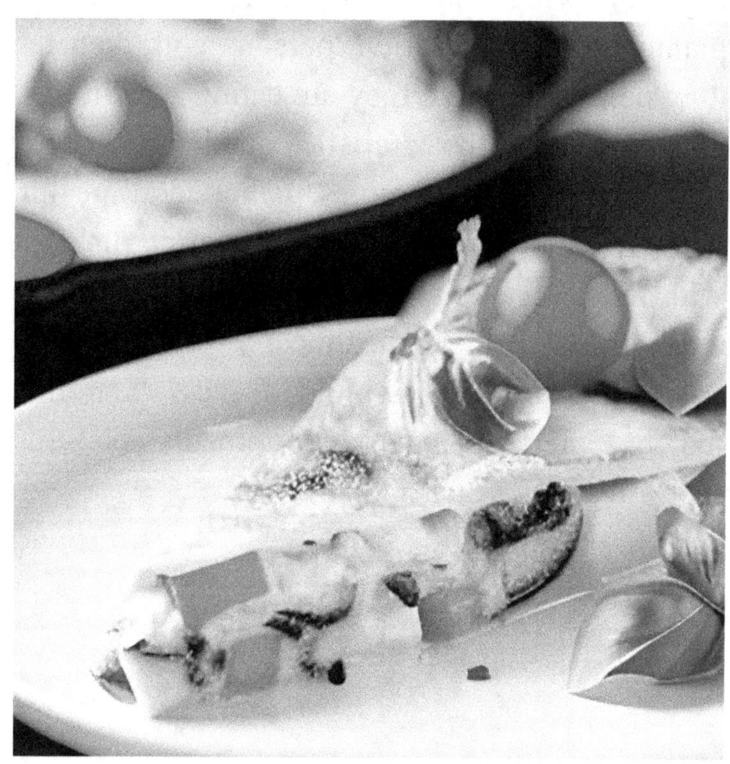

A low-carb omelet with vegetables and cheese is a tasty and healthy meal that is great for persons with diabetes. This lunch is low in carbs, rich in protein, and filled with nutrient-dense veggies. Here is a recipe for a low-carb omelet with vegetables and cheese:

Ingredients:

2 big eggs
1/4 cup chopped onion 1/4 cup chopped bell pepper
1/4 cup chopped mushrooms
1/4 cup shredded cheddar cheese
Salt and pepper to taste
Cooking spray
Instructions:

In a small bowl, mix the eggs, salt, and pepper.
Heat a non-stick skillet over medium-high heat and coat with cooking spray.
Add the onion, bell pepper, and mushrooms to the pan and simmer until soft, approximately 3-5 minutes.

Pour the egg mixture over the veggies and heat until the eggs begin to set, approximately 2-3 minutes.

Sprinkle the cheese over the top of the omelet and fold it in half.

Cook for a further 1-2 minutes, or until the cheese is melted and the eggs are cooked through.

Serve hot and enjoy!

This low-carb omelet with vegetables and cheese is a tasty and gratifying dish that can be eaten for breakfast, lunch, or supper. The combination of eggs, veggies, and cheese delivers a balanced mix of protein, fiber, and healthy fats, which may help manage blood sugar levels and enhance general health. Additionally, this meal is quick and easy to prepare, making it a great option for busy days or times when cooking is not possible.

Greek yogurt with berries and almonds

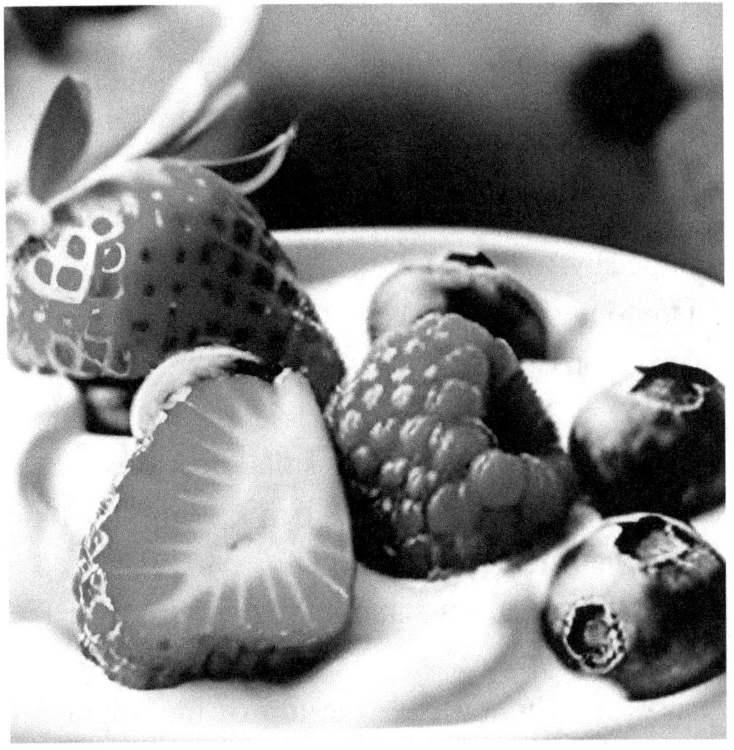

Greek yogurt with berries and almonds is a healthy and delightful snack that is great for persons with diabetes. This snack is low in carbs, rich in protein, and filled with beneficial nutrients from berries and almonds. Here is a recipe for Greek yogurt with berries and nuts:

Ingredients:

1/2 cup plain Greek yogurt
1/4 cup mixed berries (such as strawberries, blueberries, and raspberries)
1/4 cup mixed nuts (such as almonds, walnuts, and pecans)
1 tsp honey (optional)
Instructions:

Place the Greek yogurt in a small bowl.
Rinse and cut the mixed berries and sprinkle them over the yogurt.
Chop the mixed nuts and sprinkle them over the berries and yogurt.
Drizzle the honey over the top of the yogurt, if preferred.
Serve immediately and enjoy!
This Greek yogurt with berries and almonds snack is an excellent alternative for persons with diabetes who are searching for a fast and simple snack that is low in carbs and rich in protein. The Greek yogurt delivers a rich dose of protein,

which may help manage blood sugar levels and keep you feeling full and content. The mixed berries and nuts give a balanced combination of vitamins, minerals, and antioxidants, which may help enhance general health and fight against chronic illnesses. Additionally, this snack is easy to customize based on personal preferences and can be made ahead of time for a quick and convenient snack on the go.

High-fiber smoothie with avocado and spinach

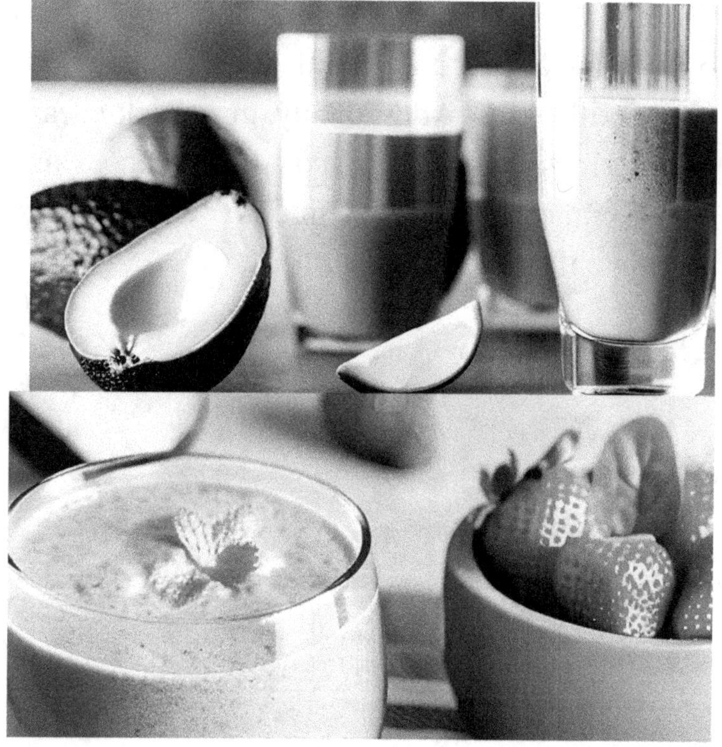

A high-fiber smoothie with avocado and spinach is a delightful and healthy drink that is great for persons with diabetes. This smoothie is low in carbs, rich in fiber, and filled with healthy fats and minerals from avocado and spinach. Here is a recipe for a high-fiber smoothie with avocado and spinach:

Ingredients:

1/2 ripe avocado
1 cup fresh spinach
1/2 cup unsweetened almond milk
1/2 cup plain Greek yogurt
1 tbsp chia seeds
1 tsp honey (optional)
Ice cubes, as required

Instructions:

Cut the avocado in half and remove the pit and peel.
In a blender, mix the avocado, spinach, almond milk, Greek yogurt, chia seeds, and honey (if using).

Blend on high speed until smooth and creamy, adding ice cubes as required to obtain desired consistency.

Pour the smoothie into a glass and serve immediately.

This high-fiber smoothie with avocado and spinach is a terrific alternative for persons with diabetes who are searching for a nutrient-dense drink that may help manage blood sugar levels and boost overall health. The avocado gives a wonderful supply of healthy fats, fiber, and vitamins, while the spinach provides a fantastic source of fiber, iron, and antioxidants. The chia seeds are also a terrific source of fiber and beneficial omega-3 fatty acids, which may help decrease inflammation and enhance heart health. Additionally, Greek yogurt provides a good source of protein, which can help keep you feeling full and satisfied. This smoothie is very simple to alter depending on personal tastes and may be prepared ahead of time for a quick and handy breakfast or snack.

Whole-grain bread with almond butter and banana

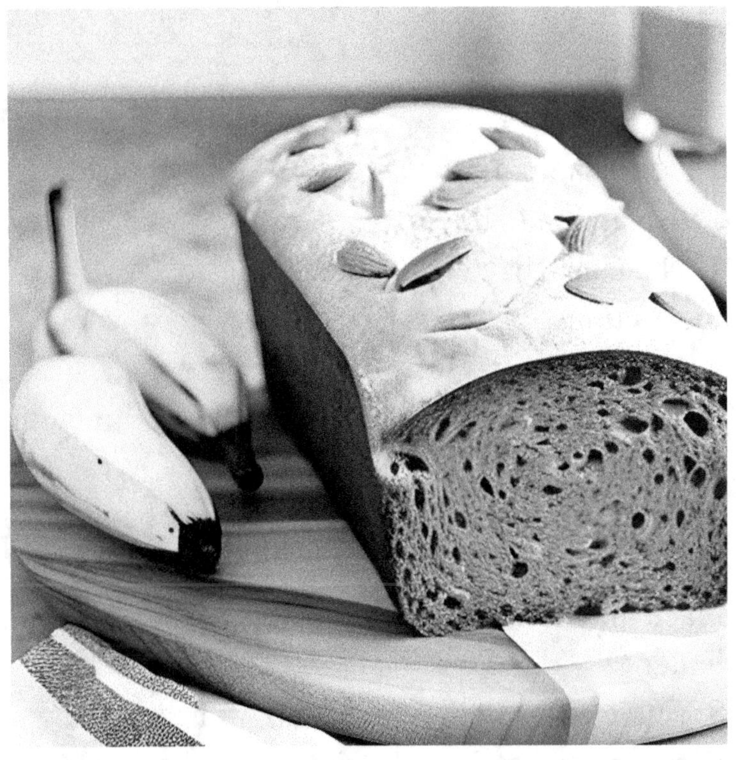

Whole-grain toast with almond butter and banana is a tasty and nutritious breakfast or snack choice that is suitable for persons with diabetes. This lunch is low in carbs, rich in fiber, and filled with beneficial nutrients from whole-grain bread, almond butter, and banana. Here is a recipe for whole-grain toast with almond butter and banana:

Ingredients:

1 piece whole-grain bread
1 tbsp almond butter
1/2 banana, sliced Cinnamon, to taste
Instructions:

Toast the piece of whole-grain bread to your chosen degree of doneness.
Spread the almond butter evenly over the toasted bread.
Place the sliced banana on top of the almond butter.
Sprinkle cinnamon over the top of the banana.
Serve immediately and enjoy!
This whole-grain toast with almond butter and banana is a terrific alternative for persons with diabetes who are searching for a quick and simple breakfast or snack that is low in carbs and

rich in fiber. The whole-grain bread is a healthy supply of fiber and complex carbs, which may help control blood sugar levels and keep you feeling full and content. Almond butter is also a terrific source of healthy fats and protein, which may help decrease inflammation and enhance heart health. The banana is a wonderful source of fiber, vitamins, and minerals, and lends a natural sweetness to the dish. Additionally, cinnamon is a great way to add flavor to the meal without adding any extra sugar or carbohydrates. This dish is very simple to alter depending on personal tastes and may be cooked ahead of time for a quick and handy breakfast or snack on the run.

Chapter Three

Lunch and Dinner Entrees

When it comes to controlling diabetes, lunch and supper may be tough meals to plan. However, there are plenty of delicious and nutritious options available for individuals with diabetes. Here are some options for lunch and supper meals that are diabetes-friendly:

Grilled Chicken Salad:

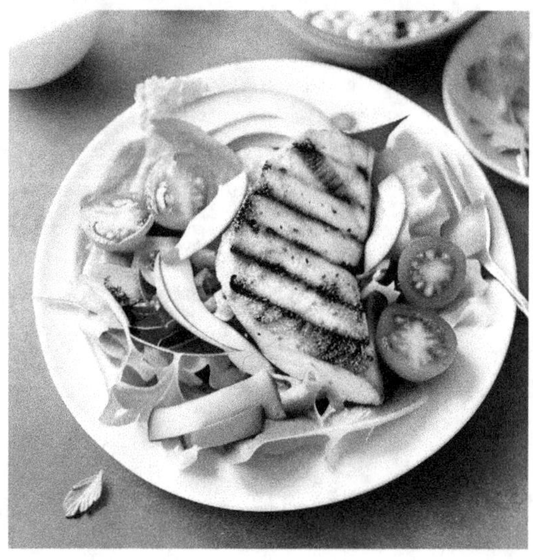

Grilled chicken salad is a terrific alternative for a diabetes-friendly lunch or supper. Simply grill some chicken breast and chop it up to add to a bed of fresh greens. Top with your favorite veggies, such as cherry tomatoes, cucumber, and bell peppers. Add a sprinkling of nuts or seeds for some crunch, then drizzle with a homemade vinaigrette prepared with olive oil and vinegar.

Turkey and Veggie Stir-Fry:

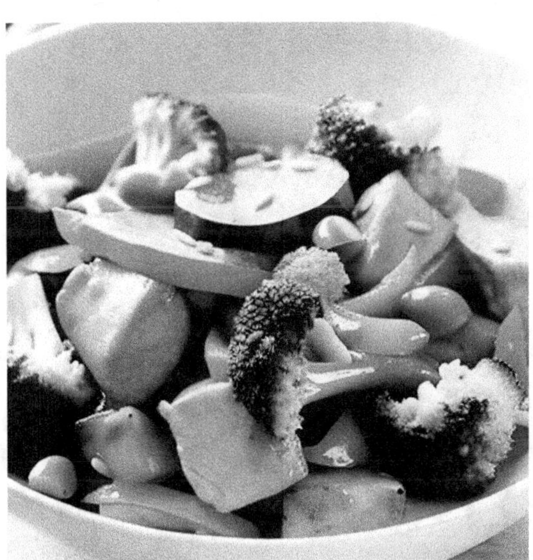

A turkey and veggie stir-fry is a terrific choice for a diabetes-friendly meal. Heat some oil in a wok or big pan, then add sliced turkey breast, along with your favorite vegetables, such as broccoli, bell peppers, and carrots. Season with some low-sodium soy sauce, garlic, and ginger. Serve over a bed of brown rice or quinoa for a satisfying and healthful supper.

Baked Salmon:

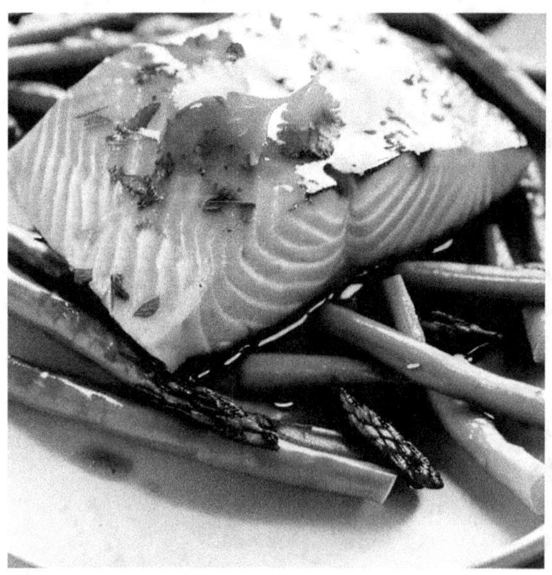

Baked salmon is a terrific choice for a diabetes-friendly meal. Simply season a salmon fillet with some herbs and spices, such as lemon juice, dill, and black pepper. Bake in the oven at 375 degrees for approximately 15-20 minutes, or until the fish is cooked through. Serve with a side of roasted vegetables, such as asparagus or Brussels sprouts, for a healthy and full supper.

Lentil Soup:

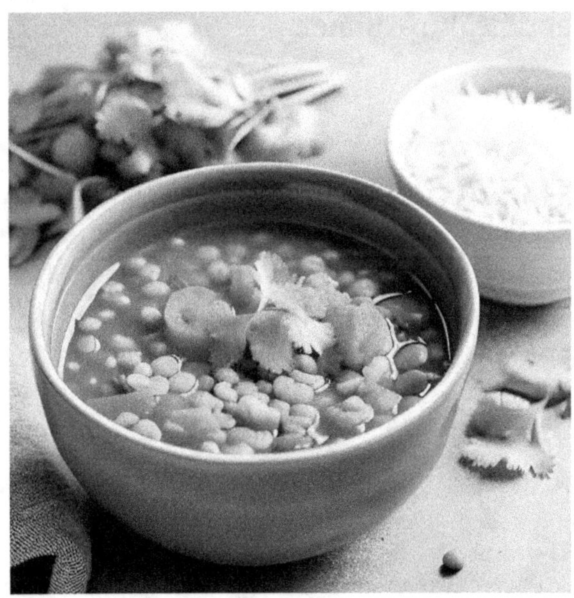

Lentil soup is a terrific alternative for a diabetes-friendly lunch or supper. Lentils are abundant in fiber and protein, making them a fantastic option for controlling blood sugar levels. Simply sauté some onions and garlic in a pot, add in some chopped carrots and celery, and cook until soft. Add in some lentils and low-sodium chicken or vegetable broth, along with some herbs and spices, such as thyme and bay leaves. Cook until the lentils are soft, then serve with a piece of whole-grain bread for a satisfying and healthy dinner.

Turkey Burger:

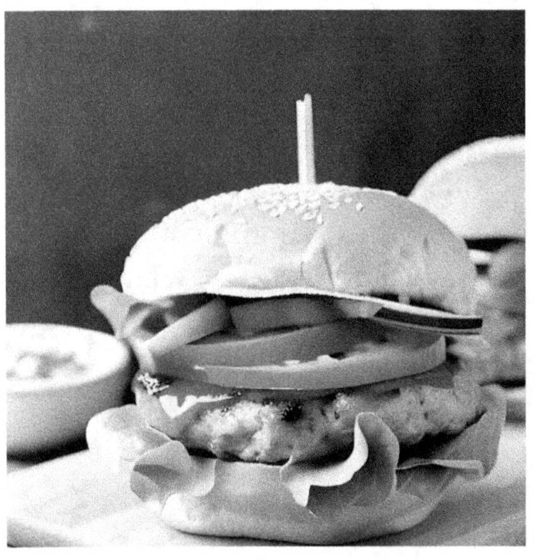

A turkey burger is a terrific choice for a diabetes-friendly lunch or supper. Simply mix ground turkey with some herbs and spices, such as garlic, onion powder, and parsley. Form into patties and grill or bake until cooked through. Serve on a loaf of whole-grain bread, then top with your favorite veggies, such as lettuce, tomato, and onion. Add a side of sweet potato fries for a satisfying and healthful supper.

there are many tasty and healthy alternatives accessible for those with diabetes when it comes to lunch and dinner dishes. The idea is to concentrate on full, nutrient-dense meals, and to reduce processed foods and added sugars. By following these rules, persons with diabetes may enjoy a broad range of tasty and healthful meals that can help manage blood sugar levels and support overall health.

Grilled salmon with roasted veggies

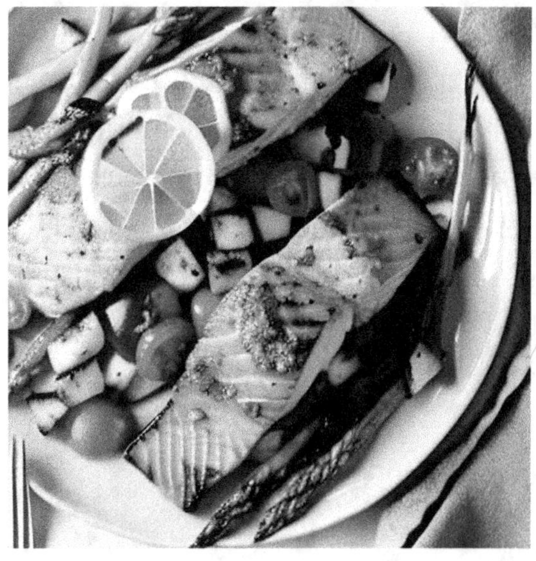

Grilled salmon with roasted veggies is a healthful and delightful alternative for persons with diabetes. Salmon is a wonderful source of protein and omega-3 fatty acids, which have been found to increase insulin sensitivity and lower the risk of heart disease. Roasted veggies are also a fantastic source of fiber and minerals, making this meal a well-rounded choice for regulating blood sugar levels.

To create this recipe, start by preheating the oven to 400 degrees Fahrenheit. Line a baking sheet with parchment paper and put aside. Next, prepare the vegetables by slicing them into bite-sized pieces. You may use your favorite veggies, such as broccoli, zucchini, bell peppers, and onions. Place the veggies on the prepared baking sheet, then drizzle with little olive oil and season with salt and pepper. Toss the veggies to coat evenly, and set the baking pan in the oven. Roast the veggies for 20-25 minutes, or until they are soft and golden brown.

While the vegetables are roasting, prepare the salmon. Heat a grill or grill pan over medium-high heat. Season the salmon with some herbs and spices, such as garlic, lemon juice, and black pepper. Grill the salmon for 3-4 minutes on each side, or until it is cooked through.

To serve, arrange the grilled salmon on a dish, and add a hearty amount of roasted veggies on the side. You may also add a squeeze of fresh lemon juice for some extra taste. This meal is both nutritious and tasty and is a fantastic alternative for persons with diabetes who wish to have a balanced and enjoyable dinner.

In addition to being a wonderful choice for persons with diabetes, grilled salmon with roasted veggies is also a fast and simple dish to make. It can be produced in about 30 minutes, making it a wonderful alternative for hectic weeknights. It may also be readily altered to fit your needs. You may mix up the veggies or spices to produce a variety of tasty and healthful dinners.

grilled salmon with roasted veggies is a healthy and delightful solution for persons with diabetes. It is rich in protein, omega-3 fatty acids, fiber, and minerals, making it a well-rounded meal that may help manage blood sugar levels and enhance overall health. With its fast and simple preparation, this dish is a fantastic alternative for busy people who want to have a nutritious and enjoyable supper.

Chicken stir-fry with brown rice

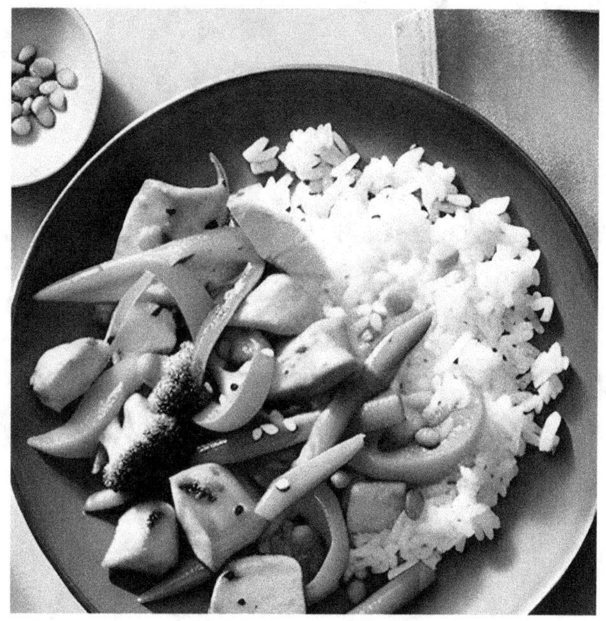

Chicken stir-fry with brown rice is a tasty and healthful dinner that is great for persons with diabetes. This meal is rich in protein, fiber, and minerals, making it a wonderful alternative for controlling blood sugar levels and supporting general health.

To create this recipe, start by cooking the brown rice according to the package directions. While the rice is cooking, prepare the chicken by slicing it into bite-sized pieces. Heat a wok or big pan over medium-high heat, and add some olive oil. Add the chicken to the pan, and cook for 3-4 minutes, or until it is cooked through.

Next, add your choice of vegetables to the wok. You may use a variety of veggies, such as bell peppers, onions, broccoli, and carrots. Cook the veggies for 3-4 minutes, or until they are soft.

To season the stir-fry, add some garlic, ginger, and soy sauce to the pan. Toss everything together to coat evenly, then heat for a further 1-2 minutes.

To serve, arrange a large portion of brown rice on a dish, then pour the chicken stir-fry on top. You may top the meal with some sliced green onions or sesame seeds for extra taste and texture.

This dish is both tasty and nutritious and is a perfect alternative for persons with diabetes who wish to have a balanced and enjoyable dinner. Brown rice is an excellent source of fiber and minerals and is a better alternative to white rice. Chicken is also an excellent source of protein, and the veggies in the stir-fry give a range of minerals and fiber.

In addition to being a nutritious alternative, chicken stir-fry with brown rice is also a flexible dinner that can be readily altered to fit your tastes. You may mix up the veggies or spices to produce a variety of tasty and healthful dinners.

chicken stir-fry with brown rice is a delightful and healthful solution for persons with diabetes. It is rich in protein, fiber, and minerals, making it a fantastic alternative for managing blood sugar levels and supporting overall health. With its fast and simple preparation and variety, this dish is a perfect alternative for busy people who want to have a nutritious and enjoyable lunch.

Turkey chili with beans and vegetables

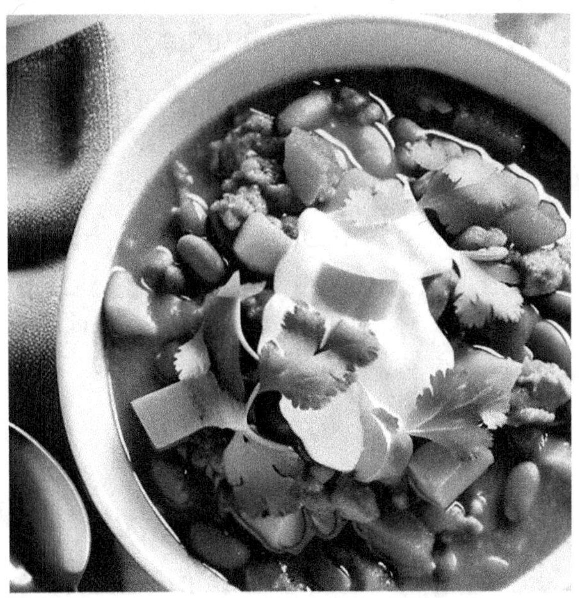

Turkey chili with beans and vegetables is a wonderful and substantial dish that is great for persons with diabetes. This meal is rich in protein, fiber, and minerals, making it a wonderful alternative for controlling blood sugar levels and supporting general health.

To cook this recipe, start by browning some ground turkey in a large saucepan over medium heat. Add chopped onions, bell peppers, and garlic to the saucepan, and simmer until the veggies are soft.

Next, add your choice of canned beans to the pot. You may use kidney beans, black beans, or a mixture of both. Rinse the beans completely before adding them to the saucepan to lower their salt level.

To add some more taste and nutrients, you may also add chopped tomatoes, tomato sauce, and a variety of seasonings to the pot. Some excellent possibilities are chili powder, cumin, paprika, and oregano. If you want your chili spicy, you may also add some cayenne pepper or hot sauce to the pot.

Simmer the chili for approximately 20-30 minutes, or until it is thick and bubbling. If you like a thicker chili, you may add some cornstarch or arrowroot powder to the saucepan.

To serve, spoon the turkey chili into bowls and garnish with some chopped fresh cilantro or green onions. You can also top the chili with some shredded cheese, plain Greek yogurt, or avocado for more taste and nutrients.

This dish is both tasty and nutritious and is a perfect alternative for persons with diabetes who wish to have a balanced and enjoyable dinner. Turkey is a lean protein source, and the beans in the chili give an excellent supply of fiber and minerals. The veggies and spices also contribute a range of nutrients and taste to the meal.

In addition to being a nutritious alternative, turkey chili with beans and vegetables is also an adaptable dish that can be readily altered to fit your tastes. You may swap up the kinds of beans or veggies to produce a range of tasty and healthful dinners.

turkey chili with beans and vegetables is a tasty and healthful solution for persons with diabetes.

It is rich in protein, fiber, and minerals, making it a fantastic alternative for managing blood sugar levels and supporting overall health. With its fast and simple preparation and variety, this dish is a perfect alternative for busy people who want to have a nutritious and enjoyable lunch.

Spinach and feta-filled chicken breast

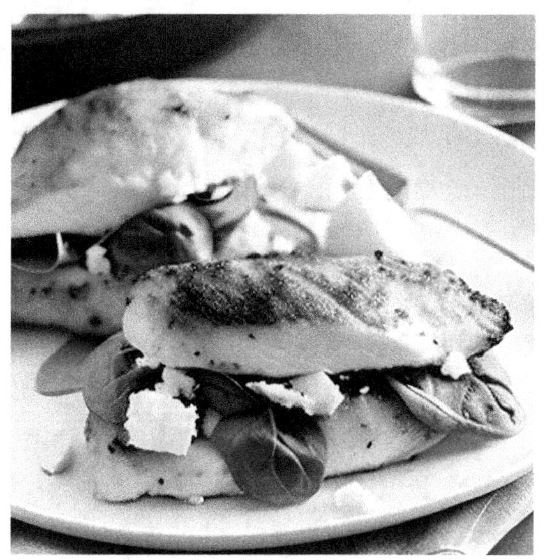

Spinach and feta-filled chicken breast is a tasty and healthful dinner that is great for persons with diabetes. This meal is rich in protein, vitamins, and minerals, making it a fantastic alternative for managing blood sugar levels and supporting general health.

To cook this recipe, start by preheating your oven to 375°F. Next, lay out your chicken breasts on a cutting board and use a sharp knife to cut a pocket into the center of each breast. Be cautious not to cut through the breast.

In a small bowl, mix some crumbled feta cheese, chopped spinach, and minced garlic. Stuff the mixture into the pockets of the chicken breasts, taking care not to overstuff them.

Next, heat some olive oil in a large oven-safe skillet over medium-high heat. Add the filled chicken breasts to the pan and cook for approximately 2-3 minutes on each side, or until they are golden brown.

Transfer the pan to the preheated oven and bake the chicken for 20-25 minutes, or until it is cooked through and no longer pink in the middle.

To serve, take the chicken from the pan and let it rest for a few minutes before slicing. You may also garnish the chicken with some chopped fresh herbs, such as parsley or basil, for extra taste and nutrients.

This dish is both tasty and nutritious and is a perfect alternative for persons with diabetes who wish to have a balanced and enjoyable dinner. The chicken offers a lean protein source, while the spinach and feta cheese give a range of vitamins and minerals.

In addition to being a nutritious alternative, spinach, and feta-filled chicken breast is also a flexible dinner that can be readily altered to fit your tastes. You may mix up the kind of cheese or veggies to produce a variety of tasty and healthful lunches.

spinach and feta-filled chicken breast is a tasty and healthful solutions for persons with diabetes. It is rich in protein, vitamins, and minerals, making it a fantastic alternative for managing blood sugar levels and supporting general health. With its fast and simple preparation and variety, this dish is a perfect alternative for busy people who want to have a nutritious and enjoyable lunch.

Chapter four

Side Dishes and Salads

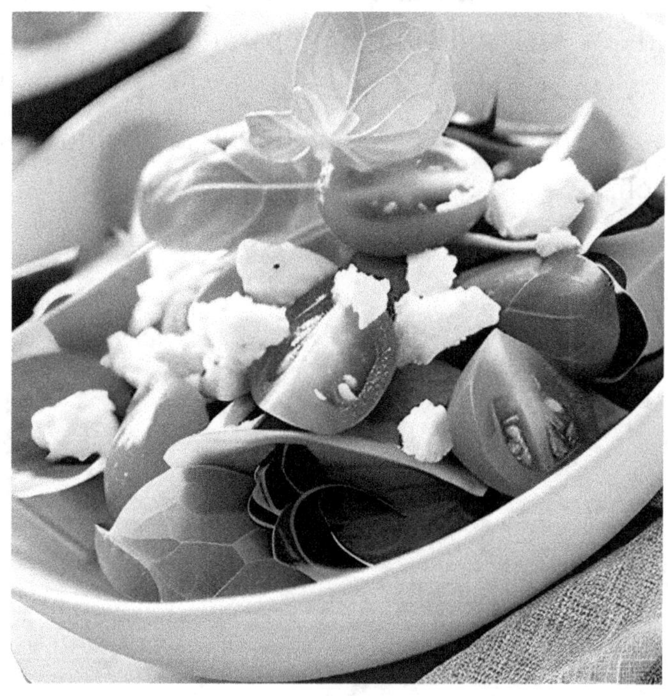

Side dishes and salads are an important element of a diabetes-friendly diet since they add crucial nutrients, fiber, and variety to meals. Here are some tasty and healthful alternatives for side dishes and salads that are great for those with diabetes.

Roasted veggies: Roasting veggies is a terrific method to bring out their natural sweetness and improve their taste. Simply toss your favorite vegetables in olive oil, sprinkle with salt and pepper, and roast in the oven at 400°F for 20-30 minutes, or until tender and lightly browned. Some great options include broccoli, cauliflower, Brussels sprouts, and sweet potatoes.

Quinoa Salad: Quinoa is a healthy and protein-packed grain that is ideal for salads. To prepare a wonderful quinoa salad, cook some quinoa according to the package guidelines, then combine it with your favorite veggies, such as diced tomatoes, cucumbers, and red onions. Drizzle with a simple vinaigrette prepared from olive oil, lemon juice, and Dijon mustard for a nutritious and tasty salad.

Greek Salad: Greek salad is a traditional Mediterranean meal that is both tasty and nutritious. To prepare a simple Greek salad, mix diced cucumbers, tomatoes, red onions, and Kalamata olives in a bowl. Top with crumbled feta cheese and a dab of olive oil and red wine vinegar for a delicious and nutritional salad.

Steamed Greens: Steamed greens, such as spinach, kale, or Swiss chard, are an excellent source of vitamins and minerals. To prepare, just wash and cut your greens, then steam them in a saucepan with a small amount of water for 2-3 minutes, or until soft. Toss with little lemon juice and a touch of salt for a simple and healthful side dish.

Roasted Chickpeas: Roasted chickpeas are a crispy and tasty snack that can also be used as a side dish. To create, sprinkle canned chickpeas in olive oil and your preferred spices, such as cumin, paprika, and garlic powder, then roast in the oven at 400°F for 20-30 minutes, or until crispy and golden brown.

Caprese Salad: Caprese salad is a simple and tasty salad composed of fresh mozzarella, tomatoes, and basil. To create, just slice the mozzarella and tomatoes, then stack them on a dish with fresh basil leaves. Drizzle with a little amount of balsamic vinegar and olive oil for a nutritious and refreshing salad.

Roasted Root Vegetables: Roasted root vegetables, such as carrots, parsnips, and beets, are an excellent source of fiber and vitamins. To prepare, cut your veggies into tiny pieces, sprinkle with olive oil, and roast in the oven at 400°F for 20-30 minutes, or until soft and gently browned.

side dishes and salads are an important element of a diabetes-friendly diet, since they give crucial nutrients and variety to meals. These nutritious and tasty alternatives are simple to make and can be adjusted to fit your tastes, making them a fantastic complement to any meal.

Roasted root vegetables

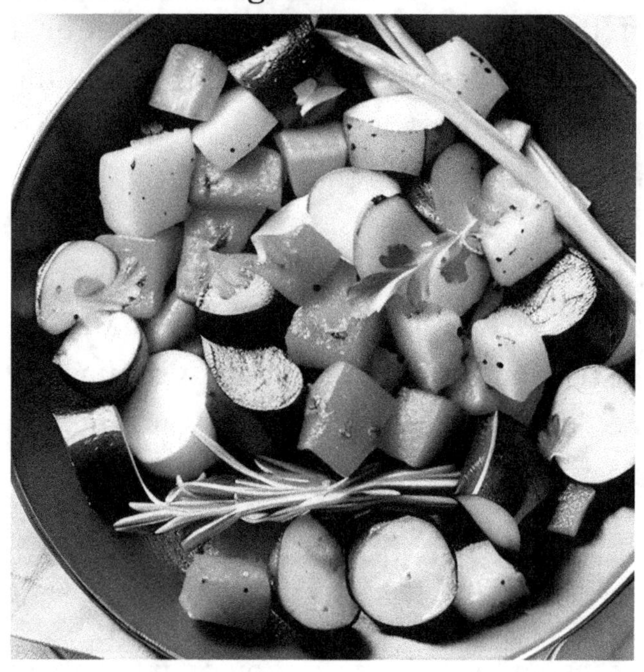

Roasted root vegetables are a wonderful and healthful complement to any meal. They are an excellent source of fiber, vitamins, and minerals, and are especially good for persons with diabetes, since they may help manage blood sugar levels.

Some of the most common root vegetables used for roasting are carrots, parsnips, beets, sweet potatoes, and turnips. These veggies are inherently sweet and grow much sweeter when roasted, giving them a wonderful alternative to high-carb and high-sugar dishes.

To create roasted root veggies, start by washing and peeling your vegetables. Cut them into equally sized pieces, so they cook evenly. Toss them with a little amount of olive oil, salt, and pepper, then lay them out on a baking sheet.

Roast the veggies in the oven at 400°F for 20-30 minutes, or until they are soft and gently browned. You may also add herbs and spices, such as rosemary, thyme, or paprika, to give extra flavor to your roasted veggies.

Roasted root vegetables may be eaten as a side dish, or added to salads, soups, or stews. They also make a terrific snack, since they are quick to cook and may be eaten hot or cold.

One of the advantages of roasted root vegetables is their adaptability. You may mix and match various kinds of veggies to produce a range of tastes and textures. For example, you may roast carrots and parsnips together for a sweet and savory combination, or roast beets and sweet potatoes for a colorful and nutrient-rich side dish.

Roasted root vegetables may also be used to produce a nutritious and full breakfast. Simply toss some roasted vegetables in a skillet with some scrambled eggs and cheese for a delicious and satisfying meal.

In addition to their excellent flavor and adaptability, roasted root vegetables are also rich in nutrients. They are a wonderful source of fiber, which may help manage blood sugar levels and enhance digestive health. They also include vitamins and minerals like vitamin A, vitamin C, potassium, and magnesium, which are crucial for sustaining general health.

Overall, roasted root veggies are a nutritious and tasty complement to any meal. They are quick to cook, adaptable, and rich in nutrients, making them a fantastic option for those with diabetes or anybody searching for a healthy and appetizing side dish.

Quinoa and black bean salad

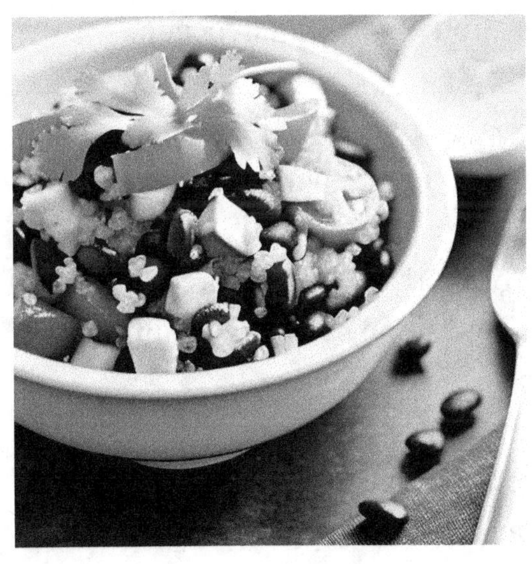

Quinoa and black bean salad is a tasty and healthy recipe that is great for anybody with diabetes or anyone trying to add more plant-based meals to their diet. This salad is rich in fiber, protein, and other necessary elements, making it a perfect option for a nutritious and fulfilling lunch or supper.

To create this salad, start by cooking the quinoa according to the package directions. While the quinoa is cooking, rinse and drain a can of black beans and chop up your vegetables. Some great options for this salad include bell peppers, cherry tomatoes, red onion, and avocado.

Once the quinoa is done, let it cool for a few minutes before mixing it with the black beans and vegetables in a large bowl. In a separate dish, mix up a basic dressing prepared with lime juice, olive oil, and some spices like cumin, chili powder, and salt.

Drizzle the dressing over the quinoa and black bean mixture and toss everything together until the salad is fully covered. You may serve the salad immediately or chill it for a few hours to allow the flavors to mingle together.

One of the beautiful things about this salad is that it can be adjusted to fit your tastes and preferences. You may add more or less of each ingredient, depending on what you have on hand or what you prefer. For example, you may add some chopped cilantro or jalapeño peppers for more flavor and fire.

This salad is not only tasty but it is also filled with vitamins. Quinoa is an excellent source of protein, fiber, and vital vitamins and minerals including iron and magnesium. Black beans are also a wonderful source of protein and fiber, and they are low in fat and calories. The veggies in this salad are rich in antioxidants, vitamins, and minerals, making this meal a terrific option for general health and well-being.

Quinoa and black bean salad is a fantastic recipe for meal prep since it can be cooked ahead of time and kept in the refrigerator for a few days. This makes it a wonderful alternative for hectic weekdays or for bringing to work or school for lunch.

quinoa and black bean salad is a nutritious and tasty dish that is great for anybody trying to add more plant-based meals to their diet. It is quick to make, customizable, and filled with critical nutrients, making it an excellent option for persons with diabetes or anybody trying to maintain a healthy and balanced diet.

Grilled asparagus with lemon and garlic

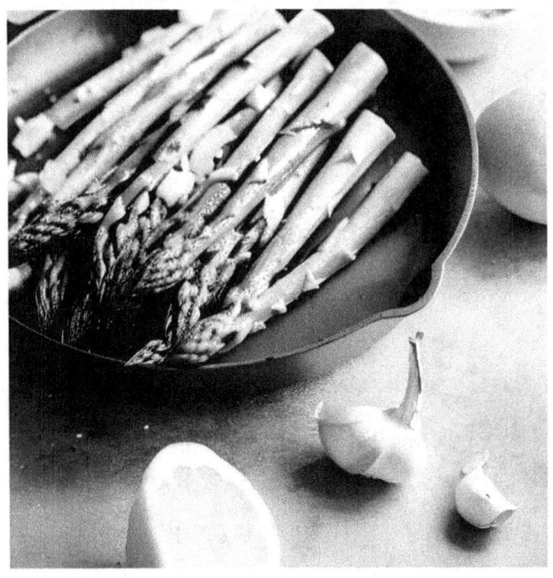

Grilled asparagus with lemon and garlic is a simple and tasty side dish that is excellent for anybody with diabetes or anyone trying to add more veggies to their diet. Asparagus is a rich source of fiber, vitamins, and minerals, making it a nutritious complement to any meal. This meal is also low in calories and carbohydrates, making it a wonderful alternative for folks who need to monitor their blood sugar levels.

To create grilled asparagus with lemon and garlic, start by cleaning and cutting the asparagus. Then, toss the asparagus with some olive oil, minced garlic, salt, and pepper. You may also add some grated lemon zest for added taste. Make sure the asparagus is fully covered with the spice mixture.

Preheat your grill to medium-high heat. Once the grill is hot, place the asparagus directly on the grates. Grill for 5-7 minutes, or until the asparagus is soft and slightly browned. You may also grill some lemon slices with the asparagus to provide some more flavor and aesthetic appeal.

Remove the asparagus from the grill and set it on a serving plate. Squeeze some fresh lemon juice over the top of the asparagus and garnish with the grilled lemon slices. Serve immediately.

Grilled asparagus with lemon and garlic is a flexible side dish that may be served with many main meals, such as grilled chicken or fish, roasted vegetables, or a simple salad. It is also an excellent alternative for summer picnics or outdoor events since it can be simply made on the grill with other foods.

This meal is not only tasty but it is also filled with nutrients. Asparagus is an excellent source of fiber, folate, vitamins A, C, E, and K, and other critical elements. Garlic is also recognized for its health advantages since it possesses anti-inflammatory and antibacterial qualities that may help decrease blood pressure and improve cholesterol levels.

grilled asparagus with lemon and garlic is a nutritious and tasty side dish that is great for anybody with diabetes or anyone trying to add more veggies to their diet. It is quick to make, full of critical nutrients, and low in calories and carbohydrates, making it a fantastic alternative for persons who need to regulate their blood sugar levels. Give this recipe a try and enjoy the fresh tastes of summer!

Kale and beet salad with goat cheese

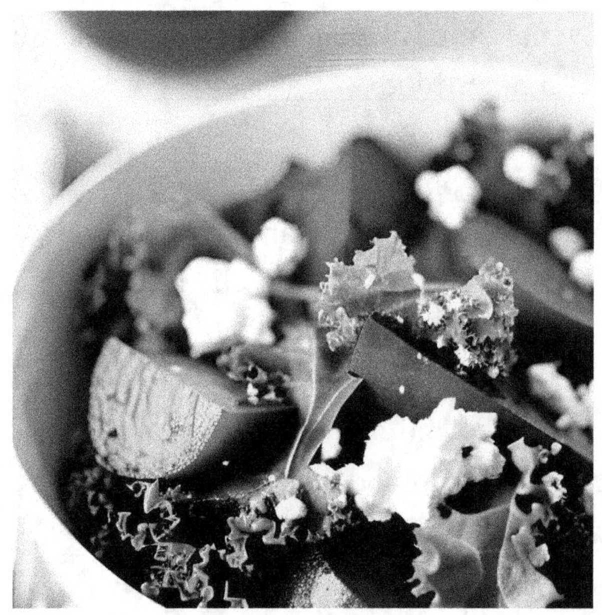

Kale and beet salad with goat cheese is a healthful and tasty recipe that is great for anybody trying to add more greens to their diet. This salad is filled with vitamins, minerals, and antioxidants, making it an excellent alternative for persons with diabetes or anybody trying to enhance their overall health.

To create this salad, start by washing and drying a bunch of kale leaves. Remove the stiff stems and slice the leaves into bite-sized pieces. Next, wash and peel a beetroot, then use a spiralizer to convert it into thin, curly strips. Alternatively, you can grate the beet using a box grater. Toss the kale and beet together in a large bowl.

Next, make the dressing. In a small bowl, stir together some olive oil, apple cider vinegar, Dijon mustard, honey, and salt & pepper. Pour the dressing over the kale and beet mixture and toss well to coat.

Finally, crumble some goat cheese over the top of the salad. You may also add some chopped nuts, such as walnuts or almonds, for some added crunch and taste.

Kale and beet salad with goat cheese is a tasty and healthy meal that is excellent for lunch or as a side dish for supper. It is low in calories and carbohydrates, making it a wonderful alternative for folks who need to maintain their blood sugar levels. Kale is a fantastic source of fiber, vitamins A, C, and K, and other critical minerals, while beets are strong in folate, potassium, and antioxidants. The goat cheese gives a creamy and tangy taste that balances the earthy tones of the kale and beets.

This salad may also be adjusted to suit your taste preferences. You may add additional veggies, such as carrots or cucumber, or switch the goat cheese for feta or blue cheese. You may also use a different kinds of greens, such as spinach or arugula if you like.

kale and beet salad with goat cheese is a healthy and tasty meal that is quick to create and filled with necessary elements. It is an excellent alternative for persons with diabetes or anybody trying to integrate more greens into their diet. Give this salad a try and enjoy the fresh and tasty mix of kale, beets, and goat cheese!

Chapter five

Snacks and Desserts

Maintaining a healthy and balanced diet is vital for controlling diabetes, but that doesn't mean you can't enjoy snacks and sweets from time to time. With a few easy replacements and conscious decisions, you can still indulge in delightful sweets while keeping your blood sugar levels in control.

Here are some suggestions for diabetes-friendly snacks and desserts:

Apple slices with almond butter: This snack is a terrific balance of protein, healthy fats, and fiber. Slice up an apple and serve it with a spoonful of almond butter for a delightful and substantial snack.

Greek yogurt with berries: Greek yogurt is an excellent source of protein and calcium, and it works nicely with fresh berries for a sweet and tangy snack. Top your yogurt with some raspberries, strawberries, or blueberries for extra fiber and antioxidants.

Hummus with vegetables: Hummus is an excellent source of protein and healthy fats, and it works nicely with fresh veggies like carrots, celery, and cucumber. This snack is quick to make and excellent for quenching the desire for something savory.

Dark chocolate: Believe it or not, dark chocolate may be a nutritious and delicious snack when taken in moderation. Choose a brand with at least 70% cacao for optimal health benefits, and keep to a modest serving size.

Baked apple with cinnamon: This simple treat is a terrific way to satisfy a sweet taste without overindulging. Slice one apple into wedges and sprinkle with cinnamon, then bake in the oven until tender and caramelized.

Berry sorbet: Sorbet is a pleasant and light dessert that may be created with fresh berries and sweetened with a natural sweetener like stevia or honey. Simply blend your berries with some water and sweetener, then freeze until solid.

Chia seed pudding: Chia seeds are a terrific source of fiber and healthy fats, and they form a great basis for a pudding-like treat. Mix chia seeds with some unsweetened almond milk and a natural sweetener like maple syrup or honey, then let it rest in the fridge until thick and creamy.

By picking snacks and treats that are rich in fiber, protein, and healthy fats, you may fulfill your desires and maintain stable blood sugar levels. It's also vital to pay attention to portion sizes and avoid meals that are heavy in processed sugars and carbohydrates.

with a little imagination and some wise decisions, it's feasible to enjoy great snacks and sweets while controlling diabetes. By concentrating on whole, nutrient-dense foods and reducing processed and sugary foods, you may maintain a healthy and balanced diet that promotes your overall health and wellness.

Apple slices with peanut butter

Apple slices with peanut butter are a traditional snack combo that is both tasty and wholesome. Apples are abundant in fiber, antioxidants, and vitamins, while peanut butter provides a fantastic source of healthy fats and protein. Together, they produce a pleasant and full snack that may help manage blood sugar levels and prevent cravings.

To create this snack, just slice up an apple and apply some peanut butter to each piece. You may choose a natural peanut butter that is free from added sugars and oils, or you can create your own by mixing peanuts in a food processor until smooth.

One of the nice things about this snack is that it is adaptable and adjustable. You may add various toppings to your apple slices, such as sliced bananas, raisins, or chopped almonds. You may also sprinkle some cinnamon or cocoa powder on top for extra taste and antioxidants.

When picking an apple, choose a kind that is lower in sugar, such as Granny Smith or Honeycrisp. These types are less prone to trigger a quick surge in blood sugar levels than sweeter kinds like Gala or Red Delicious.

It's crucial to remember that although this snack is healthful, it is still necessary to pay attention to portion amounts. Nuts and nut jars of butter are heavy in calories and fat, so it's better to keep to a serving size of 1-2 teaspoons of peanut butter per apple. This will guarantee that you are receiving the advantages of this food without overdoing it on calories and fat.

Overall, apple slices with peanut butter are a tasty and nutritious snack that may help control diabetes and fulfill your desires. By selecting nutrient-dense foods and being cautious of portion sizes, you may enjoy this snack as part of a balanced and nutritious diet.

Hummus and vegetable sticks

Hummus and vegetable sticks make for a delightful and healthful snack that is great for controlling diabetes. Hummus is produced with chickpeas, which are a fantastic source of fiber and protein, while veggies give a range of vitamins and minerals.

To create this snack, you will need a jar of hummus and a variety of fresh veggies, such as carrots, celery, cucumber, and bell peppers. Simply slice the vegetables into sticks and dip them into the hummus for a tasty and nutritious snack.

One of the beautiful things about this snack is that it is incredibly adaptable. You may add other varieties of hummus, such as roasted red pepper, garlic, or lemon, to mix up the taste. You may also add additional toppings to the hummus, such as olives or sliced tomatoes, for extra texture and taste.

When picking a hummus, aim for a brand that is minimal in added sugars and preservatives. You may also create your hummus at home using canned chickpeas, tahini, garlic, lemon juice, and olive oil.

The veggies you pick to combine with the hummus are equally significant. Opt for vegetables that are low in carbohydrates and high in fiber, such as carrots, celery, and bell peppers. These veggies will help control blood sugar levels and keep you feeling full and content.

It's crucial to remember that although this snack is healthy, it's still necessary to pay attention to portion quantities. Hummus is heavy in calories and fat, therefore it's better to keep to a serving size of 2-3 tablespoons every snack. The veggies are minimal in calories, so you may have as many as you wish.

Overall, hummus and vegetable sticks are delightful and healthful snacks that may help control diabetes and boost overall health. By selecting nutrient-dense foods and being cautious of portion sizes, you may enjoy this snack as part of a balanced and nutritious diet.

Dark chocolate with almond clusters

Dark chocolate and almond clusters are delightful and fulfilling snack that is great for treating diabetes. Dark chocolate is rich in antioxidants and flavonoids, which may help enhance insulin sensitivity and manage blood sugar levels. Almonds are also an excellent option since they are packed with protein, fiber, and healthy fats.

To create this snack, you will need dark chocolate chips, raw almonds, and a sprinkle of sea salt. Begin by toasting the almonds in a dry pan over medium heat until they are lightly toasted and aromatic. Remove from heat and put aside.

Next, melt the dark chocolate chips in a double boiler or microwave, stirring frequently to prevent burning. Once melted, add the toasted almonds and stir to combine.

Using a spoon or a cookie scoop, put the chocolate and almond mixture onto a baking sheet lined with parchment paper. Sprinkle a sprinkle of sea salt over each cluster, if preferred.

Allow the clusters to cool and harden in the refrigerator for about 30 minutes. Once cooled, you can store them in an airtight container at room temperature for up to one week.

It's crucial to remember that although this snack is healthful, it's still rich in calories and fat. It's preferable to keep to a serving size of 1-2 clusters for every snack. Pairing this snack with a source of protein or fiber, such as a handful of raw vegetables or a cooked egg, will help balance blood sugar levels and keep you feeling full and content.

general, dark chocolate and almond clusters are delightful and healthful snacks that may help control diabetes and boost general health. By selecting nutrient-dense foods and being cautious of portion sizes, you may enjoy this snack as part of a balanced and nutritious diet.

Berry and yogurt parfait

A berry and yogurt parfait is a nutritious and delightful snack or dessert that may be eaten as part of a diabetes-friendly diet. This parfait is packed with fiber, protein, and antioxidants, which may help manage blood sugar levels and enhance general health.

To prepare this parfait, you will need Greek yogurt, mixed berries, granola, and honey. Begin by spooning a layer of Greek yogurt into a transparent glass or parfait dish. Next, add a layer of mixed berries, such as strawberries, blueberries, and raspberries. You may use fresh or frozen berries for this dish.

Sprinkle a layer of granola over the berries, then continue the layers until you reach the top of the glass. Drizzle a tiny bit of honey over the top of the parfait, if preferred.

Greek yogurt is a terrific option for this dish since it is strong in protein and low in sugar. Berries are also an excellent option since they are packed with fiber and antioxidants. Granola may give extra fiber and crunch, but be careful to pick a low-sugar kind.

This parfait may be eaten as a nutritious snack or dessert, and it can be adjusted to fit your tastes. You may mix up the sorts of berries, add a layer of chopped nuts, or swap out the granola for another type of crunchy topping.

It's crucial to remember that although this parfait is nutritious, it's still vital to control portion sizes and pick nutrient-dense meals. Aim for a serving size of 1/2 to 1 cup, and pair this snack with a source of protein or healthy fat, such as a boiled egg or a handful of almonds.

general, a berry and yogurt parfait is a delightful and healthful snack that may help control diabetes and boost general health. By selecting nutrient-dense foods and being cautious of portion sizes, you may enjoy this snack as part of a balanced and nutritious diet.

Chapter Six

Conclusion

Maintaining a diabetes-friendly diet is vital for regulating blood sugar levels and supporting overall health. Here are some key points to keep in mind when planning meals:

Choose nutrient-dense foods: Focus on foods that are rich in fiber, protein, and healthy fats, such as fruits, vegetables, whole grains, lean protein sources, and nuts and seeds.

Limit refined carbohydrates and added sugars: Avoid highly processed meals and sugary beverages, which may trigger blood sugar rises.

Portion control: Be conscious of portion sizes and strive for a balanced meal that contains a supply of protein, healthy fats, and complex carbohydrates.

Meal planning and preparation: Plan and prepare healthy meals and snacks in advance to minimize impulsive eating or reaching for bad choices.

Hydration: Stay hydrated by drinking lots of water and minimizing sugary drinks.

Regular monitoring: Regularly check blood sugar levels and collaborate with a healthcare practitioner to change meal plans as required.

By following these essential concepts, persons with diabetes may maintain a nutritious and balanced diet that promotes their overall health and well-being.

Additional resources for diabetes management

In addition to adopting a diabetic-friendly diet, there are various resources available for controlling diabetes and supporting general health. Here are some extra sites to consider:

Diabetes education programs: Many healthcare professionals provide diabetes education programs to assist patients to learn more about managing their illness, including food planning, exercise, and medication administration.

Physical activity: Regular exercise may help regulate blood sugar levels and boost overall health. Consider working with a healthcare physician or licensed personal trainer to establish a safe and effective workout regimen.

Diabetes support groups: Joining a support group may give emotional support and help people connect with others who are going through similar circumstances.

Continuous glucose monitoring: Continuous glucose monitoring (CGM) devices may give real-time information about blood sugar levels and help users make better-educated choices regarding food and medication management.

Telehealth services: Telehealth services, such as virtual visits with a healthcare practitioner, may offer convenient and accessible care for patients with diabetes.

Medication treatment: In addition to diet and exercise, medication management may be important for certain patients with diabetes. Work together with a healthcare physician to design a suitable pharmaceutical regimen.

Overall, treating diabetes involves a multi-faceted strategy that includes food, exercise, medication management, and support from healthcare practitioners and loved ones. By using the services available and keeping proactive about controlling their disease, persons with diabetes may have healthy and meaningful lives.

Final thoughts and encouragement.

Living with diabetes may be tough, but it's essential to realize that it's possible to keep a healthy and satisfying lifestyle with the correct treatment. By adopting a diabetic-friendly diet, remaining physically active, and using the services available, persons with diabetes may take control of their health and avoid problems.

It's essential to remember that everyone's path with diabetes is unique, and there may be ups and downs along the road. However, with the right mindset and support, it's possible to overcome challenges and achieve long-term success.

If you're dealing with controlling diabetes, know that you're not alone. Reach out to your healthcare practitioner or a support group for help and encouragement. Remember to appreciate your victories, no matter how minor, and be nice to yourself along the journey.

Living with diabetes might be a daily hardship, but it's also a chance to prioritize your health and well-being. With the correct mentality and tools, you can take charge of your health and live a happy and fulfilled life.

www.ingramcontent.com/pod-product-compliance
Lightning Source LLC
Chambersburg PA
CBHW051832250726
48659CB00005B/1805